# RUNCRASTINATION
## (noun)

having a long list of things to do but going for a long run instead

# RUNNING / JOGGING LOG

YEAR      MONTH

| DATE | DISTANCE | TIME | PACE | HR | REST HR | RUN TYPE | SHOES | NOTES |
|------|----------|------|------|----|---------|----------|-------|-------|
|  |  |  |  |  |  |  |  |  |
|  |  |  |  |  |  |  |  |  |
|  |  |  |  |  |  |  |  |  |
|  |  |  |  |  |  |  |  |  |
|  |  |  |  |  |  |  |  |  |
|  |  |  |  |  |  |  |  |  |
|  |  |  |  |  |  |  |  |  |
|  |  |  |  |  |  |  |  |  |
|  |  |  |  |  |  |  |  |  |
|  |  |  |  |  |  |  |  |  |
|  |  |  |  |  |  |  |  |  |
|  |  |  |  |  |  |  |  |  |
|  |  |  |  |  |  |  |  |  |
|  |  |  |  |  |  |  |  |  |
|  |  |  |  |  |  |  |  |  |
|  |  |  |  |  |  |  |  |  |
|  |  |  |  |  |  |  |  |  |
| DATE | DISTANCE | TIME | PACE | HR | REST HR | RUN TYPE | SHOES | NOTES |

# RUNNING / JOGGING LOG

YEAR             MONTH

| DATE | DISTANCE | TIME | PACE | HR | REST HR | RUN TYPE | SHOES | | NOTES |
|------|----------|------|------|----|---------|----------|-------|--|-------|
| | | | | | | | | | |
| | | | | | | | | | |
| | | | | | | | | | |
| | | | | | | | | | |
| | | | | | | | | | |
| | | | | | | | | | |
| | | | | | | | | | |
| | | | | | | | | | |
| | | | | | | | | | |
| | | | | | | | | | |
| | | | | | | | | | |
| | | | | | | | | | |
| | | | | | | | | | |
| | | | | | | | | | |
| | | | | | | | | | |
| | | | | | | | | | |
| | | | | | | | | | |
| | | | | | | | | | |
| | | | | | | | | | |
| | | | | | | | | | |

# RUNNING / JOGGING LOG

YEAR ............ MONTH ............

| DATE | DISTANCE | TIME | PACE | HR | REST HR | RUN TYPE | SHOES | NOTES |
|------|----------|------|------|----|---------|----------|-------|-------|
| | | | | | | | | |
| | | | | | | | | |
| | | | | | | | | |
| | | | | | | | | |
| | | | | | | | | |
| | | | | | | | | |
| | | | | | | | | |
| | | | | | | | | |
| | | | | | | | | |
| | | | | | | | | |
| | | | | | | | | |
| | | | | | | | | |
| | | | | | | | | |
| | | | | | | | | |
| | | | | | | | | |
| | | | | | | | | |
| | | | | | | | | |
| | | | | | | | | |

| DATE | DISTANCE | TIME | PACE | HR | REST HR | RUN TYPE | SHOES | NOTES |
|------|----------|------|------|----|---------|----------|-------|-------|

# RUNNING / JOGGING LOG

YEAR ___________ MONTH ___________

| DATE | DISTANCE | TIME | PACE | HR | REST HR | RUN TYPE | SHOES | NOTES |
|------|----------|------|------|-----|---------|----------|-------|-------|
| | | | | | | | | |
| | | | | | | | | |
| | | | | | | | | |
| | | | | | | | | |
| | | | | | | | | |
| | | | | | | | | |
| | | | | | | | | |
| | | | | | | | | |
| | | | | | | | | |
| | | | | | | | | |
| | | | | | | | | |
| | | | | | | | | |
| | | | | | | | | |
| | | | | | | | | |
| | | | | | | | | |
| | | | | | | | | |
| | | | | | | | | |
| | | | | | | | | |
| | | | | | | | | |
| | | | | | | | | |

# RUNNING / JOGGING LOG

YEAR            MONTH

| DATE | DISTANCE | TIME | PACE | HR | REST HR | RUN TYPE | SHOES | NOTES |
|------|----------|------|------|----|---------|----------|-------|-------|
|      |          |      |      |    |         |          |       |       |

YEAR            MONTH

| DATE | DISTANCE | TIME | PACE | HR | REST HR | RUN TYPE | SHOES | NOTES |
|------|----------|------|------|----|---------|----------|-------|-------|
|      |          |      |      |    |         |          |       |       |

# RUNNING / JOGGING LOG

YEAR              MONTH

| DATE | DISTANCE | TIME | PACE | HR | REST HR | RUN TYPE | SHOES | | NOTES |
|------|----------|------|------|-----|---------|----------|-------|--|-------|
| | | | | | | | | | |
| | | | | | | | | | |
| | | | | | | | | | |
| | | | | | | | | | |
| | | | | | | | | | |
| | | | | | | | | | |
| | | | | | | | | | |
| | | | | | | | | | |
| | | | | | | | | | |
| | | | | | | | | | |
| | | | | | | | | | |
| | | | | | | | | | |
| | | | | | | | | | |
| | | | | | | | | | |
| | | | | | | | | | |
| | | | | | | | | | |
| | | | | | | | | | |
| | | | | | | | | | |
| | | | | | | | | | |
| | | | | | | | | | |

# RUNNING / JOGGING LOG

YEAR _______ MONTH _______

| DATE | DISTANCE | TIME | PACE | HR | REST HR | RUN TYPE | SHOES | NOTES |
|------|----------|------|------|----|---------|----------|-------|-------|
|      |          |      |      |    |         |          |       |       |

YEAR _______ MONTH _______

| DATE | DISTANCE | TIME | PACE | HR | REST HR | RUN TYPE | SHOES | NOTES |
|------|----------|------|------|----|---------|----------|-------|-------|
|      |          |      |      |    |         |          |       |       |

# RUNNING / JOGGING LOG

YEAR        MONTH

| DATE | DISTANCE | TIME | PACE | HR | REST HR | RUN TYPE | SHOES | | NOTES |
|------|----------|------|------|----|---------|----------|-------|--|-------|
|  |  |  |  |  |  |  |  |  |  |
|  |  |  |  |  |  |  |  |  |  |
|  |  |  |  |  |  |  |  |  |  |
|  |  |  |  |  |  |  |  |  |  |
|  |  |  |  |  |  |  |  |  |  |
|  |  |  |  |  |  |  |  |  |  |
|  |  |  |  |  |  |  |  |  |  |
|  |  |  |  |  |  |  |  |  |  |
|  |  |  |  |  |  |  |  |  |  |
|  |  |  |  |  |  |  |  |  |  |
|  |  |  |  |  |  |  |  |  |  |
|  |  |  |  |  |  |  |  |  |  |
|  |  |  |  |  |  |  |  |  |  |
|  |  |  |  |  |  |  |  |  |  |
|  |  |  |  |  |  |  |  |  |  |
|  |  |  |  |  |  |  |  |  |  |

# RUNNING / JOGGING LOG

YEAR            MONTH

| DATE | DISTANCE | TIME | PACE | HR | REST HR | RUN TYPE | SHOES | NOTES |
|------|----------|------|------|-----|---------|----------|-------|-------|
|      |          |      |      |     |         |          |       |       |

# RUNNING / JOGGING LOG

YEAR ________  MONTH ________

| DATE | DISTANCE | TIME | PACE | HR | REST HR | RUN TYPE | SHOES | NOTES |
|------|----------|------|------|----|---------|----------|-------|-------|
|      |          |      |      |    |         |          |       |       |
|      |          |      |      |    |         |          |       |       |
|      |          |      |      |    |         |          |       |       |
|      |          |      |      |    |         |          |       |       |
|      |          |      |      |    |         |          |       |       |
|      |          |      |      |    |         |          |       |       |
|      |          |      |      |    |         |          |       |       |
|      |          |      |      |    |         |          |       |       |
|      |          |      |      |    |         |          |       |       |
|      |          |      |      |    |         |          |       |       |
|      |          |      |      |    |         |          |       |       |
|      |          |      |      |    |         |          |       |       |
|      |          |      |      |    |         |          |       |       |
|      |          |      |      |    |         |          |       |       |
|      |          |      |      |    |         |          |       |       |

| DATE | DISTANCE | TIME | PACE | HR | REST HR | RUN TYPE | SHOES | NOTES |
|------|----------|------|------|----|---------|----------|-------|-------|
|      |          |      |      |    |         |          |       |       |

# RUNNING / JOGGING LOG

YEAR      MONTH

| DATE | DISTANCE | TIME | PACE | HR | REST HR | RUN TYPE | SHOES | NOTES |
|------|----------|------|------|-----|---------|----------|-------|-------|
|      |          |      |      |     |         |          |       |       |

| DATE | DISTANCE | TIME | PACE | HR | REST HR | RUN TYPE | SHOES | NOTES |
|------|----------|------|------|-----|---------|----------|-------|-------|
|      |          |      |      |     |         |          |       |       |

# RUNNING / JOGGING LOG

YEAR __________ MONTH __________

| DATE | DISTANCE | TIME | PACE | HR | REST HR | RUN TYPE | SHOES | NOTES |
|------|----------|------|------|----|---------|----------|-------|-------|
|      |          |      |      |    |         |          |       |       |

YEAR __________ MONTH __________

# RUNNING / JOGGING LOG

YEAR          MONTH

| DATE | DISTANCE | TIME | PACE | HR | REST HR | RUN TYPE | SHOES | NOTES |
|------|----------|------|------|----|---------|----------|-------|-------|
|      |          |      |      |    |         |          |       |       |

| DATE | DISTANCE | TIME | PACE | HR | REST HR | RUN TYPE | SHOES | NOTES |
|------|----------|------|------|----|---------|----------|-------|-------|
|      |          |      |      |    |         |          |       |       |

# RUNNING / JOGGING LOG

YEAR ______  MONTH ______

| DATE | DISTANCE | TIME | PACE | HR | REST HR | RUN TYPE | SHOES | NOTES |
|------|----------|------|------|----|---------|----------|-------|-------|
|  |  |  |  |  |  |  |  |  |
|  |  |  |  |  |  |  |  |  |
|  |  |  |  |  |  |  |  |  |
|  |  |  |  |  |  |  |  |  |
|  |  |  |  |  |  |  |  |  |
|  |  |  |  |  |  |  |  |  |
|  |  |  |  |  |  |  |  |  |
|  |  |  |  |  |  |  |  |  |
|  |  |  |  |  |  |  |  |  |
|  |  |  |  |  |  |  |  |  |
|  |  |  |  |  |  |  |  |  |
|  |  |  |  |  |  |  |  |  |
|  |  |  |  |  |  |  |  |  |
|  |  |  |  |  |  |  |  |  |
|  |  |  |  |  |  |  |  |  |

| DATE | DISTANCE | TIME | PACE | HR | REST HR | RUN TYPE | SHOES | NOTES |
|------|----------|------|------|----|---------|----------|-------|-------|
|  |  |  |  |  |  |  |  |  |

# RUNNING / JOGGING LOG

YEAR __________ MONTH __________

| DATE | DISTANCE | TIME | PACE | HR | REST HR | RUN TYPE | SHOES | NOTES |
|------|----------|------|------|----|---------|----------|-------|-------|
|      |          |      |      |    |         |          |       |       |
|      |          |      |      |    |         |          |       |       |
|      |          |      |      |    |         |          |       |       |
|      |          |      |      |    |         |          |       |       |
|      |          |      |      |    |         |          |       |       |
|      |          |      |      |    |         |          |       |       |
|      |          |      |      |    |         |          |       |       |
|      |          |      |      |    |         |          |       |       |
|      |          |      |      |    |         |          |       |       |
|      |          |      |      |    |         |          |       |       |
|      |          |      |      |    |         |          |       |       |
|      |          |      |      |    |         |          |       |       |
|      |          |      |      |    |         |          |       |       |
|      |          |      |      |    |         |          |       |       |
|      |          |      |      |    |         |          |       |       |
|      |          |      |      |    |         |          |       |       |
|      |          |      |      |    |         |          |       |       |
|      |          |      |      |    |         |          |       |       |
|      |          |      |      |    |         |          |       |       |
|      |          |      |      |    |         |          |       |       |

| DATE | DISTANCE | TIME | PACE | HR | REST HR | RUN TYPE | SHOES | NOTES |
|------|----------|------|------|----|---------|----------|-------|-------|

# RUNNING / JOGGING LOG

YEAR          MONTH

| DATE | DISTANCE | TIME | PACE | HR | REST HR | RUN TYPE | SHOES | | NOTES |
|------|----------|------|------|----|---------|----------|-------|--|-------|
| | | | | | | | | | |
| | | | | | | | | | |
| | | | | | | | | | |
| | | | | | | | | | |
| | | | | | | | | | |
| | | | | | | | | | |
| | | | | | | | | | |
| | | | | | | | | | |
| | | | | | | | | | |
| | | | | | | | | | |
| | | | | | | | | | |
| | | | | | | | | | |
| | | | | | | | | | |
| | | | | | | | | | |
| | | | | | | | | | |
| | | | | | | | | | |
| | | | | | | | | | |
| | | | | | | | | | |
| | | | | | | | | | |

| DATE | DISTANCE | TIME | PACE | HR | REST HR | RUN TYPE | SHOES | | NOTES |
|------|----------|------|------|----|---------|----------|-------|--|-------|
| | | | | | | | | | |

# RUNNING / JOGGING LOG

YEAR __________ MONTH __________

| DATE | DISTANCE | TIME | PACE | HR | REST HR | RUN TYPE | SHOES | | NOTES |
|------|----------|------|------|-----|---------|----------|-------|--|-------|
|      |          |      |      |     |         |          |       |  |       |

| DATE | DISTANCE | TIME | PACE | HR | REST HR | RUN TYPE | SHOES | | NOTES |
|------|----------|------|------|-----|---------|----------|-------|--|-------|
|      |          |      |      |     |         |          |       |  |       |

# RUNNING / JOGGING LOG

YEAR ____________ MONTH ____________

| DATE | DISTANCE | TIME | PACE | HR | REST HR | RUN TYPE | SHOES | | NOTES |
|------|----------|------|------|----|---------|----------|-------|--|-------|
| | | | | | | | | | |
| | | | | | | | | | |
| | | | | | | | | | |
| | | | | | | | | | |
| | | | | | | | | | |
| | | | | | | | | | |
| | | | | | | | | | |
| | | | | | | | | | |
| | | | | | | | | | |
| | | | | | | | | | |
| | | | | | | | | | |
| | | | | | | | | | |
| | | | | | | | | | |
| | | | | | | | | | |
| | | | | | | | | | |
| | | | | | | | | | |
| | | | | | | | | | |
| | | | | | | | | | |
| | | | | | | | | | |

# RUNNING / JOGGING LOG

YEAR              MONTH

| DATE | DISTANCE | TIME | PACE | HR | REST HR | RUN TYPE | SHOES | NOTES |
|------|----------|------|------|----|---------|----------|-------|-------|
|      |          |      |      |    |         |          |       |       |
|      |          |      |      |    |         |          |       |       |
|      |          |      |      |    |         |          |       |       |
|      |          |      |      |    |         |          |       |       |
|      |          |      |      |    |         |          |       |       |
|      |          |      |      |    |         |          |       |       |
|      |          |      |      |    |         |          |       |       |
|      |          |      |      |    |         |          |       |       |
|      |          |      |      |    |         |          |       |       |
|      |          |      |      |    |         |          |       |       |
|      |          |      |      |    |         |          |       |       |
|      |          |      |      |    |         |          |       |       |
|      |          |      |      |    |         |          |       |       |
|      |          |      |      |    |         |          |       |       |
|      |          |      |      |    |         |          |       |       |
|      |          |      |      |    |         |          |       |       |
|      |          |      |      |    |         |          |       |       |
|      |          |      |      |    |         |          |       |       |
|      |          |      |      |    |         |          |       |       |

YEAR              MONTH

| DATE | DISTANCE | TIME | PACE | HR | REST HR | RUN TYPE | SHOES | NOTES |
|------|----------|------|------|----|---------|----------|-------|-------|
|      |          |      |      |    |         |          |       |       |
|      |          |      |      |    |         |          |       |       |

# RUNNING / JOGGING LOG

YEAR _______  MONTH _______

| DATE | DISTANCE | TIME | PACE | HR | REST HR | RUN TYPE | SHOES | NOTES |
|------|----------|------|------|----|---------|----------|-------|-------|
|      |          |      |      |    |         |          |       |       |

| DATE | DISTANCE | TIME | PACE | HR | REST HR | RUN TYPE | SHOES | NOTES |
|------|----------|------|------|----|---------|----------|-------|-------|
|      |          |      |      |    |         |          |       |       |

# RUNNING / JOGGING LOG

YEAR　　　　MONTH

| DATE | DISTANCE | TIME | PACE | HR | REST HR | RUN TYPE | SHOES | NOTES |
|------|----------|------|------|-----|---------|----------|-------|-------|
|  |  |  |  |  |  |  |  |  |

| DATE | DISTANCE | TIME | PACE | HR | REST HR | RUN TYPE | SHOES | NOTES |
|------|----------|------|------|-----|---------|----------|-------|-------|
|  |  |  |  |  |  |  |  |  |

# RUNNING / JOGGING LOG

YEAR __________ MONTH __________

| DATE | DISTANCE | TIME | PACE | HR | REST HR | RUN TYPE | SHOES | NOTES |
|------|----------|------|------|-----|---------|----------|-------|-------|
|      |          |      |      |     |         |          |       |       |
|      |          |      |      |     |         |          |       |       |
|      |          |      |      |     |         |          |       |       |
|      |          |      |      |     |         |          |       |       |
|      |          |      |      |     |         |          |       |       |
|      |          |      |      |     |         |          |       |       |
|      |          |      |      |     |         |          |       |       |
|      |          |      |      |     |         |          |       |       |
|      |          |      |      |     |         |          |       |       |
|      |          |      |      |     |         |          |       |       |
|      |          |      |      |     |         |          |       |       |
|      |          |      |      |     |         |          |       |       |
|      |          |      |      |     |         |          |       |       |
|      |          |      |      |     |         |          |       |       |
|      |          |      |      |     |         |          |       |       |
|      |          |      |      |     |         |          |       |       |
|      |          |      |      |     |         |          |       |       |
|      |          |      |      |     |         |          |       |       |

# RUNNING / JOGGING LOG

YEAR        MONTH

| DATE | DISTANCE | TIME | PACE | HR | REST HR | RUN TYPE | SHOES | NOTES |
|------|----------|------|------|----|---------|----------|-------|-------|
|      |          |      |      |    |         |          |       |       |

| DATE | DISTANCE | TIME | PACE | HR | REST HR | RUN TYPE | SHOES | NOTES |
|------|----------|------|------|----|---------|----------|-------|-------|
|      |          |      |      |    |         |          |       |       |

# RUNNING / JOGGING LOG

YEAR ___________ MONTH ___________

| DATE | DISTANCE | TIME | PACE | HR | REST HR | RUN TYPE | SHOES | NOTES |
|------|----------|------|------|----|---------|----------|-------|-------|
| | | | | | | | | |
| | | | | | | | | |
| | | | | | | | | |
| | | | | | | | | |
| | | | | | | | | |
| | | | | | | | | |
| | | | | | | | | |
| | | | | | | | | |
| | | | | | | | | |
| | | | | | | | | |
| | | | | | | | | |
| | | | | | | | | |
| | | | | | | | | |
| | | | | | | | | |
| | | | | | | | | |
| | | | | | | | | |
| | | | | | | | | |
| | | | | | | | | |
| | | | | | | | | |

| DATE | DISTANCE | TIME | PACE | HR | REST HR | RUN TYPE | SHOES | NOTES |
|------|----------|------|------|----|---------|----------|-------|-------|

# RUNNING / JOGGING LOG

YEAR __________ MONTH __________

| DATE | DISTANCE | TIME | PACE | HR | REST HR | RUN TYPE | SHOES | NOTES |
|------|----------|------|------|----|---------|----------|-------|-------|
|      |          |      |      |    |         |          |       |       |
|      |          |      |      |    |         |          |       |       |
|      |          |      |      |    |         |          |       |       |
|      |          |      |      |    |         |          |       |       |
|      |          |      |      |    |         |          |       |       |
|      |          |      |      |    |         |          |       |       |
|      |          |      |      |    |         |          |       |       |
|      |          |      |      |    |         |          |       |       |
|      |          |      |      |    |         |          |       |       |
|      |          |      |      |    |         |          |       |       |

| DATE | DISTANCE | TIME | PACE | HR | REST HR | RUN TYPE | SHOES | NOTES |
|------|----------|------|------|----|---------|----------|-------|-------|

# RUNNING / JOGGING LOG

YEAR        MONTH

| DATE | DISTANCE | TIME | PACE | HR | REST HR | RUN TYPE | SHOES | NOTES |
|------|----------|------|------|----|---------|----------|-------|-------|
|      |          |      |      |    |         |          |       |       |

# RUNNING / JOGGING LOG

YEAR            MONTH

| DATE | DISTANCE | TIME | PACE | HR | REST HR | RUN TYPE | SHOES | NOTES |
|------|----------|------|------|----|---------|----------|-------|-------|
|      |          |      |      |    |         |          |       |       |

| DATE | DISTANCE | TIME | PACE | HR | REST HR | RUN TYPE | SHOES | NOTES |
|------|----------|------|------|----|---------|----------|-------|-------|
|      |          |      |      |    |         |          |       |       |

# RUNNING / JOGGING LOG

YEAR _______ MONTH _______

| DATE | DISTANCE | TIME | PACE | HR | REST HR | RUN TYPE | SHOES | NOTES |
|------|----------|------|------|----|---------|----------|-------|-------|
| | | | | | | | | |
| | | | | | | | | |
| | | | | | | | | |
| | | | | | | | | |
| | | | | | | | | |
| | | | | | | | | |
| | | | | | | | | |
| | | | | | | | | |
| | | | | | | | | |
| | | | | | | | | |
| | | | | | | | | |
| | | | | | | | | |
| | | | | | | | | |
| | | | | | | | | |
| | | | | | | | | |
| | | | | | | | | |

# RUNNING / JOGGING LOG

YEAR              MONTH

| DATE | DISTANCE | TIME | PACE | HR | REST HR | RUN TYPE | SHOES | NOTES |
|------|----------|------|------|----|---------|----------|-------|-------|
|      |          |      |      |    |         |          |       |       |
|      |          |      |      |    |         |          |       |       |
|      |          |      |      |    |         |          |       |       |
|      |          |      |      |    |         |          |       |       |
|      |          |      |      |    |         |          |       |       |
|      |          |      |      |    |         |          |       |       |
|      |          |      |      |    |         |          |       |       |
|      |          |      |      |    |         |          |       |       |
|      |          |      |      |    |         |          |       |       |
|      |          |      |      |    |         |          |       |       |
|      |          |      |      |    |         |          |       |       |
|      |          |      |      |    |         |          |       |       |
|      |          |      |      |    |         |          |       |       |
|      |          |      |      |    |         |          |       |       |
|      |          |      |      |    |         |          |       |       |
|      |          |      |      |    |         |          |       |       |

YEAR              MONTH

| DATE | DISTANCE | TIME | PACE | HR | REST HR | RUN TYPE | SHOES | NOTES |
|------|----------|------|------|----|---------|----------|-------|-------|
|      |          |      |      |    |         |          |       |       |
|      |          |      |      |    |         |          |       |       |

# RUNNING / JOGGING LOG

YEAR          MONTH

| DATE | DISTANCE | TIME | PACE | HR | REST HR | RUN TYPE | SHOES | NOTES |
|------|----------|------|------|----|---------|----------|-------|-------|
|      |          |      |      |    |         |          |       |       |

YEAR          MONTH

| DATE | DISTANCE | TIME | PACE | HR | REST HR | RUN TYPE | SHOES | NOTES |
|------|----------|------|------|----|---------|----------|-------|-------|
|      |          |      |      |    |         |          |       |       |

# RUNNING / JOGGING LOG

YEAR _______  MONTH _______

| DATE | DISTANCE | TIME | PACE | HR | REST HR | RUN TYPE | SHOES | NOTES |
|------|----------|------|------|----|---------|----------|-------|-------|
|      |          |      |      |    |         |          |       |       |
|      |          |      |      |    |         |          |       |       |
|      |          |      |      |    |         |          |       |       |
|      |          |      |      |    |         |          |       |       |
|      |          |      |      |    |         |          |       |       |
|      |          |      |      |    |         |          |       |       |
|      |          |      |      |    |         |          |       |       |
|      |          |      |      |    |         |          |       |       |
|      |          |      |      |    |         |          |       |       |
|      |          |      |      |    |         |          |       |       |

| DATE | DISTANCE | TIME | PACE | HR | REST HR | RUN TYPE | SHOES | NOTES |
|------|----------|------|------|----|---------|----------|-------|-------|

# RUNNING / JOGGING LOG

YEAR      MONTH

| DATE | DISTANCE | TIME | PACE | HR | REST HR | RUN TYPE | SHOES | NOTES |
|------|----------|------|------|----|---------|----------|-------|-------|
|  |  |  |  |  |  |  |  |  |
|  |  |  |  |  |  |  |  |  |
|  |  |  |  |  |  |  |  |  |
|  |  |  |  |  |  |  |  |  |
|  |  |  |  |  |  |  |  |  |
|  |  |  |  |  |  |  |  |  |
|  |  |  |  |  |  |  |  |  |
|  |  |  |  |  |  |  |  |  |
|  |  |  |  |  |  |  |  |  |
|  |  |  |  |  |  |  |  |  |
|  |  |  |  |  |  |  |  |  |
|  |  |  |  |  |  |  |  |  |
|  |  |  |  |  |  |  |  |  |
|  |  |  |  |  |  |  |  |  |
|  |  |  |  |  |  |  |  |  |
|  |  |  |  |  |  |  |  |  |
|  |  |  |  |  |  |  |  |  |
|  |  |  |  |  |  |  |  |  |
|  |  |  |  |  |  |  |  |  |
|  |  |  |  |  |  |  |  |  |
|  |  |  |  |  |  |  |  |  |
|  |  |  |  |  |  |  |  |  |
| DATE | DISTANCE | TIME | PACE | HR | REST HR | RUN TYPE | SHOES | NOTES |
|  |  |  |  |  |  |  |  |  |

# RUNNING / JOGGING LOG

YEAR　　　　MONTH

| DATE | DISTANCE | TIME | PACE | HR | REST HR | RUN TYPE | SHOES | NOTES |
|------|----------|------|------|-----|---------|----------|-------|-------|
|      |          |      |      |     |         |          |       |       |
|      |          |      |      |     |         |          |       |       |
|      |          |      |      |     |         |          |       |       |
|      |          |      |      |     |         |          |       |       |
|      |          |      |      |     |         |          |       |       |
|      |          |      |      |     |         |          |       |       |
|      |          |      |      |     |         |          |       |       |
|      |          |      |      |     |         |          |       |       |
|      |          |      |      |     |         |          |       |       |
|      |          |      |      |     |         |          |       |       |
|      |          |      |      |     |         |          |       |       |
|      |          |      |      |     |         |          |       |       |
|      |          |      |      |     |         |          |       |       |
|      |          |      |      |     |         |          |       |       |
|      |          |      |      |     |         |          |       |       |
|      |          |      |      |     |         |          |       |       |
|      |          |      |      |     |         |          |       |       |
| DATE | DISTANCE | TIME | PACE | HR | REST HR | RUN TYPE | SHOES | NOTES |
|      |          |      |      |     |         |          |       |       |

# RUNNING / JOGGING LOG

YEAR ________   MONTH ________

| DATE | DISTANCE | TIME | PACE | HR | REST HR | RUN TYPE | SHOES | NOTES |
|------|----------|------|------|----|---------|----------|-------|-------|
|      |          |      |      |    |         |          |       |       |
|      |          |      |      |    |         |          |       |       |
|      |          |      |      |    |         |          |       |       |
|      |          |      |      |    |         |          |       |       |
|      |          |      |      |    |         |          |       |       |
|      |          |      |      |    |         |          |       |       |
|      |          |      |      |    |         |          |       |       |
|      |          |      |      |    |         |          |       |       |
|      |          |      |      |    |         |          |       |       |
|      |          |      |      |    |         |          |       |       |
|      |          |      |      |    |         |          |       |       |
|      |          |      |      |    |         |          |       |       |

| DATE | DISTANCE | TIME | PACE | HR | REST HR | RUN TYPE | SHOES | NOTES |
|------|----------|------|------|----|---------|----------|-------|-------|

# RUNNING / JOGGING LOG

YEAR       MONTH

| DATE | DISTANCE | TIME | PACE | HR | REST HR | RUN TYPE | SHOES | | NOTES |
|------|----------|------|------|----|---------|----------|-------|---|-------|
|  |  |  |  |  |  |  |  |  |  |
|  |  |  |  |  |  |  |  |  |  |
|  |  |  |  |  |  |  |  |  |  |
|  |  |  |  |  |  |  |  |  |  |
|  |  |  |  |  |  |  |  |  |  |
|  |  |  |  |  |  |  |  |  |  |
|  |  |  |  |  |  |  |  |  |  |
|  |  |  |  |  |  |  |  |  |  |
|  |  |  |  |  |  |  |  |  |  |
|  |  |  |  |  |  |  |  |  |  |
|  |  |  |  |  |  |  |  |  |  |
|  |  |  |  |  |  |  |  |  |  |
|  |  |  |  |  |  |  |  |  |  |
|  |  |  |  |  |  |  |  |  |  |
|  |  |  |  |  |  |  |  |  |  |
|  |  |  |  |  |  |  |  |  |  |
|  |  |  |  |  |  |  |  |  |  |
|  |  |  |  |  |  |  |  |  |  |
|  |  |  |  |  |  |  |  |  |  |

YEAR       MONTH

| DATE | DISTANCE | TIME | PACE | HR | REST HR | RUN TYPE | SHOES | | NOTES |
|------|----------|------|------|----|---------|----------|-------|---|-------|
|  |  |  |  |  |  |  |  |  |  |

# RUNNING / JOGGING LOG

YEAR            MONTH

| DATE | DISTANCE | TIME | PACE | HR | REST HR | RUN TYPE | SHOES | | NOTES |
|------|----------|------|------|----|---------|----------|-------|--|-------|
| | | | | | | | | | |
| | | | | | | | | | |
| | | | | | | | | | |
| | | | | | | | | | |
| | | | | | | | | | |
| | | | | | | | | | |
| | | | | | | | | | |
| | | | | | | | | | |
| | | | | | | | | | |
| | | | | | | | | | |
| | | | | | | | | | |
| | | | | | | | | | |
| | | | | | | | | | |
| | | | | | | | | | |
| | | | | | | | | | |
| | | | | | | | | | |
| | | | | | | | | | |
| | | | | | | | | | |
| DATE | DISTANCE | TIME | PACE | HR | REST HR | RUN TYPE | SHOES | | NOTES |
| | | | | | | | | | |

# RUNNING / JOGGING LOG

YEAR      MONTH

| DATE | DISTANCE | TIME | PACE | HR | REST HR | RUN TYPE | SHOES | NOTES |
|------|----------|------|------|----|---------|----------|-------|-------|
|      |          |      |      |    |         |          |       |       |
|      |          |      |      |    |         |          |       |       |
|      |          |      |      |    |         |          |       |       |
|      |          |      |      |    |         |          |       |       |
|      |          |      |      |    |         |          |       |       |
|      |          |      |      |    |         |          |       |       |
|      |          |      |      |    |         |          |       |       |
|      |          |      |      |    |         |          |       |       |
|      |          |      |      |    |         |          |       |       |
|      |          |      |      |    |         |          |       |       |

| DATE | DISTANCE | TIME | PACE | HR | REST HR | RUN TYPE | SHOES | NOTES |
|------|----------|------|------|----|---------|----------|-------|-------|

# RUNNING / JOGGING LOG

YEAR          MONTH

| DATE | DISTANCE | TIME | PACE | HR | REST HR | RUN TYPE | SHOES | NOTES |
|------|----------|------|------|-----|---------|----------|-------|-------|
|      |          |      |      |     |         |          |       |       |

# RUNNING / JOGGING LOG

YEAR      MONTH

| DATE | DISTANCE | TIME | PACE | HR | REST HR | RUN TYPE | SHOES | NOTES |
|------|----------|------|------|----|---------|----------|-------|-------|
|      |          |      |      |    |         |          |       |       |

| DATE | DISTANCE | TIME | PACE | HR | REST HR | RUN TYPE | SHOES | NOTES |
|------|----------|------|------|----|---------|----------|-------|-------|
|      |          |      |      |    |         |          |       |       |

# RUNNING / JOGGING LOG

YEAR ............ MONTH ............

| DATE | DISTANCE | TIME | PACE | HR | REST HR | RUN TYPE | SHOES | NOTES |
|------|----------|------|------|-----|---------|----------|-------|-------|
|      |          |      |      |     |         |          |       |       |
|      |          |      |      |     |         |          |       |       |
|      |          |      |      |     |         |          |       |       |
|      |          |      |      |     |         |          |       |       |
|      |          |      |      |     |         |          |       |       |
|      |          |      |      |     |         |          |       |       |
|      |          |      |      |     |         |          |       |       |
|      |          |      |      |     |         |          |       |       |
|      |          |      |      |     |         |          |       |       |
|      |          |      |      |     |         |          |       |       |
|      |          |      |      |     |         |          |       |       |
|      |          |      |      |     |         |          |       |       |
|      |          |      |      |     |         |          |       |       |
|      |          |      |      |     |         |          |       |       |
|      |          |      |      |     |         |          |       |       |
|      |          |      |      |     |         |          |       |       |
|      |          |      |      |     |         |          |       |       |

| DATE | DISTANCE | TIME | PACE | HR | REST HR | RUN TYPE | SHOES | NOTES |
|------|----------|------|------|-----|---------|----------|-------|-------|

# RUNNING / JOGGING LOG

YEAR ___________  MONTH ___________

| DATE | DISTANCE | TIME | PACE | HR | REST HR | RUN TYPE | SHOES | NOTES |
|------|----------|------|------|----|---------|----------|-------|-------|
|      |          |      |      |    |         |          |       |       |

| DATE | DISTANCE | TIME | PACE | HR | REST HR | RUN TYPE | SHOES | NOTES |
|------|----------|------|------|----|---------|----------|-------|-------|
|      |          |      |      |    |         |          |       |       |

# RUNNING / JOGGING LOG

YEAR ________  MONTH ________

| DATE | DISTANCE | TIME | PACE | HR | REST HR | RUN TYPE | SHOES | NOTES |
|------|----------|------|------|----|---------|----------|-------|-------|
|  |  |  |  |  |  |  |  |  |
|  |  |  |  |  |  |  |  |  |
|  |  |  |  |  |  |  |  |  |
|  |  |  |  |  |  |  |  |  |
|  |  |  |  |  |  |  |  |  |
|  |  |  |  |  |  |  |  |  |
|  |  |  |  |  |  |  |  |  |
|  |  |  |  |  |  |  |  |  |
|  |  |  |  |  |  |  |  |  |
|  |  |  |  |  |  |  |  |  |
|  |  |  |  |  |  |  |  |  |
|  |  |  |  |  |  |  |  |  |
|  |  |  |  |  |  |  |  |  |
|  |  |  |  |  |  |  |  |  |
|  |  |  |  |  |  |  |  |  |
|  |  |  |  |  |  |  |  |  |

| DATE | DISTANCE | TIME | PACE | HR | REST HR | RUN TYPE | SHOES | NOTES |
|------|----------|------|------|----|---------|----------|-------|-------|
|  |  |  |  |  |  |  |  |  |
|  |  |  |  |  |  |  |  |  |

# RUNNING / JOGGING LOG

YEAR ____________ MONTH ____________

| DATE | DISTANCE | TIME | PACE | HR | REST HR | RUN TYPE | SHOES | NOTES |
|------|----------|------|------|-----|---------|----------|-------|-------|
|      |          |      |      |     |         |          |       |       |
|      |          |      |      |     |         |          |       |       |
|      |          |      |      |     |         |          |       |       |
|      |          |      |      |     |         |          |       |       |
|      |          |      |      |     |         |          |       |       |
|      |          |      |      |     |         |          |       |       |
|      |          |      |      |     |         |          |       |       |
|      |          |      |      |     |         |          |       |       |
|      |          |      |      |     |         |          |       |       |
|      |          |      |      |     |         |          |       |       |
|      |          |      |      |     |         |          |       |       |
|      |          |      |      |     |         |          |       |       |
|      |          |      |      |     |         |          |       |       |
|      |          |      |      |     |         |          |       |       |
|      |          |      |      |     |         |          |       |       |
|      |          |      |      |     |         |          |       |       |
|      |          |      |      |     |         |          |       |       |
|      |          |      |      |     |         |          |       |       |

| DATE | DISTANCE | TIME | PACE | HR | REST HR | RUN TYPE | SHOES | NOTES |
|------|----------|------|------|-----|---------|----------|-------|-------|

# RUNNING / JOGGING LOG

YEAR          MONTH

| DATE | DISTANCE | TIME | PACE | HR | REST HR | RUN TYPE | SHOES | | NOTES |
|------|----------|------|------|-----|---------|----------|-------|---|-------|
| | | | | | | | | | |
| | | | | | | | | | |
| | | | | | | | | | |
| | | | | | | | | | |
| | | | | | | | | | |
| | | | | | | | | | |
| | | | | | | | | | |
| | | | | | | | | | |
| | | | | | | | | | |
| | | | | | | | | | |
| | | | | | | | | | |
| | | | | | | | | | |
| | | | | | | | | | |
| | | | | | | | | | |
| | | | | | | | | | |
| | | | | | | | | | |
| DATE | DISTANCE | TIME | PACE | HR | REST HR | RUN TYPE | SHOES | | NOTES |

# RUNNING / JOGGING LOG

YEAR        MONTH

| DATE | DISTANCE | TIME | PACE | HR | REST HR | RUN TYPE | SHOES | NOTES |
|------|----------|------|------|-----|---------|----------|-------|-------|
|  |  |  |  |  |  |  |  |  |

| DATE | DISTANCE | TIME | PACE | HR | REST HR | RUN TYPE | SHOES | NOTES |
|------|----------|------|------|-----|---------|----------|-------|-------|
|  |  |  |  |  |  |  |  |  |

# RUNNING / JOGGING LOG

YEAR      MONTH

| DATE | DISTANCE | TIME | PACE | HR | REST HR | RUN TYPE | SHOES | NOTES |
|------|----------|------|------|----|---------|----------|-------|-------|
|  |  |  |  |  |  |  |  |  |

| DATE | DISTANCE | TIME | PACE | HR | REST HR | RUN TYPE | SHOES | NOTES |
|------|----------|------|------|----|---------|----------|-------|-------|
|  |  |  |  |  |  |  |  |  |

# RUNNING / JOGGING LOG

YEAR ________  MONTH ________

| DATE | DISTANCE | TIME | PACE | HR | REST HR | RUN TYPE | SHOES | NOTES |
|------|----------|------|------|----|---------|----------|-------|-------|
|      |          |      |      |    |         |          |       |       |

| DATE | DISTANCE | TIME | PACE | HR | REST HR | RUN TYPE | SHOES | NOTES |
|------|----------|------|------|----|---------|----------|-------|-------|
|      |          |      |      |    |         |          |       |       |

# RUNNING / JOGGING LOG

YEAR _______ MONTH _______

| DATE | DISTANCE | TIME | PACE | HR | REST HR | RUN TYPE | SHOES | NOTES |
|------|----------|------|------|----|---------|----------|-------|-------|
|  |  |  |  |  |  |  |  |  |
|  |  |  |  |  |  |  |  |  |
|  |  |  |  |  |  |  |  |  |
|  |  |  |  |  |  |  |  |  |
|  |  |  |  |  |  |  |  |  |

| DATE | DISTANCE | TIME | PACE | HR | REST HR | RUN TYPE | SHOES | NOTES |
|------|----------|------|------|----|---------|----------|-------|-------|
|  |  |  |  |  |  |  |  |  |
|  |  |  |  |  |  |  |  |  |

# RUNNING / JOGGING LOG

YEAR      MONTH

| DATE | DISTANCE | TIME | PACE | HR | REST HR | RUN TYPE | SHOES | NOTES |
|------|----------|------|------|----|---------|----------|-------|-------|
|      |          |      |      |    |         |          |       |       |

# RUNNING / JOGGING LOG

YEAR ______     MONTH ______

| DATE | DISTANCE | TIME | PACE | HR | REST HR | RUN TYPE | SHOES | | NOTES |
|------|----------|------|------|----|---------|----------|-------|--|-------|
|  |  |  |  |  |  |  |  |  |  |
|  |  |  |  |  |  |  |  |  |  |
|  |  |  |  |  |  |  |  |  |  |
|  |  |  |  |  |  |  |  |  |  |
|  |  |  |  |  |  |  |  |  |  |
|  |  |  |  |  |  |  |  |  |  |
|  |  |  |  |  |  |  |  |  |  |
|  |  |  |  |  |  |  |  |  |  |
|  |  |  |  |  |  |  |  |  |  |
|  |  |  |  |  |  |  |  |  |  |
|  |  |  |  |  |  |  |  |  |  |
|  |  |  |  |  |  |  |  |  |  |
|  |  |  |  |  |  |  |  |  |  |
|  |  |  |  |  |  |  |  |  |  |
|  |  |  |  |  |  |  |  |  |  |
|  |  |  |  |  |  |  |  |  |  |
|  |  |  |  |  |  |  |  |  |  |
|  |  |  |  |  |  |  |  |  |  |

| DATE | DISTANCE | TIME | PACE | HR | REST HR | RUN TYPE | SHOES | | NOTES |
|------|----------|------|------|----|---------|----------|-------|--|-------|

# RUNNING / JOGGING LOG

YEAR      MONTH

| DATE | DISTANCE | TIME | PACE | HR | REST HR | RUN TYPE | SHOES | | NOTES |
|------|----------|------|------|----|---------|----------|-------|--|-------|
| | | | | | | | | | |
| | | | | | | | | | |
| | | | | | | | | | |
| | | | | | | | | | |
| | | | | | | | | | |
| | | | | | | | | | |
| | | | | | | | | | |
| | | | | | | | | | |
| | | | | | | | | | |
| | | | | | | | | | |
| | | | | | | | | | |
| | | | | | | | | | |
| | | | | | | | | | |
| | | | | | | | | | |
| | | | | | | | | | |
| | | | | | | | | | |
| | | | | | | | | | |
| | | | | | | | | | |
| | | | | | | | | | |
| DATE | DISTANCE | TIME | PACE | HR | REST HR | RUN TYPE | SHOES | | NOTES |
| | | | | | | | | | |

# RUNNING / JOGGING LOG

YEAR      MONTH

| DATE | DISTANCE | TIME | PACE | HR | REST HR | RUN TYPE | SHOES | NOTES |
|---|---|---|---|---|---|---|---|---|
|  |  |  |  |  |  |  |  |  |
|  |  |  |  |  |  |  |  |  |
|  |  |  |  |  |  |  |  |  |
|  |  |  |  |  |  |  |  |  |
|  |  |  |  |  |  |  |  |  |
|  |  |  |  |  |  |  |  |  |
|  |  |  |  |  |  |  |  |  |
|  |  |  |  |  |  |  |  |  |
|  |  |  |  |  |  |  |  |  |
|  |  |  |  |  |  |  |  |  |
|  |  |  |  |  |  |  |  |  |
|  |  |  |  |  |  |  |  |  |
|  |  |  |  |  |  |  |  |  |
|  |  |  |  |  |  |  |  |  |
|  |  |  |  |  |  |  |  |  |
|  |  |  |  |  |  |  |  |  |
|  |  |  |  |  |  |  |  |  |
|  |  |  |  |  |  |  |  |  |

| DATE | DISTANCE | TIME | PACE | HR | REST HR | RUN TYPE | SHOES | NOTES |
|---|---|---|---|---|---|---|---|---|
|  |  |  |  |  |  |  |  |  |
|  |  |  |  |  |  |  |  |  |

# RUNNING / JOGGING LOG

YEAR          MONTH

| DATE | DISTANCE | TIME | PACE | HR | REST HR | RUN TYPE | SHOES | NOTES |
|------|----------|------|------|----|---------|----------|-------|-------|
|      |          |      |      |    |         |          |       |       |

YEAR          MONTH

| DATE | DISTANCE | TIME | PACE | HR | REST HR | RUN TYPE | SHOES | NOTES |
|------|----------|------|------|----|---------|----------|-------|-------|
|      |          |      |      |    |         |          |       |       |

# RUNNING / JOGGING LOG

YEAR        MONTH

| DATE | DISTANCE | TIME | PACE | HR | REST HR | RUN TYPE | SHOES | | NOTES |
|------|----------|------|------|-----|---------|----------|-------|---|-------|
|  |  |  |  |  |  |  |  |  |  |
|  |  |  |  |  |  |  |  |  |  |
|  |  |  |  |  |  |  |  |  |  |
|  |  |  |  |  |  |  |  |  |  |
|  |  |  |  |  |  |  |  |  |  |
|  |  |  |  |  |  |  |  |  |  |
|  |  |  |  |  |  |  |  |  |  |
|  |  |  |  |  |  |  |  |  |  |
|  |  |  |  |  |  |  |  |  |  |
|  |  |  |  |  |  |  |  |  |  |
|  |  |  |  |  |  |  |  |  |  |
|  |  |  |  |  |  |  |  |  |  |
|  |  |  |  |  |  |  |  |  |  |
|  |  |  |  |  |  |  |  |  |  |
|  |  |  |  |  |  |  |  |  |  |
|  |  |  |  |  |  |  |  |  |  |
|  |  |  |  |  |  |  |  |  |  |
|  |  |  |  |  |  |  |  |  |  |

| DATE | DISTANCE | TIME | PACE | HR | REST HR | RUN TYPE | SHOES | | NOTES |
|------|----------|------|------|-----|---------|----------|-------|---|-------|

# RUNNING / JOGGING LOG

YEAR          MONTH

| DATE | DISTANCE | TIME | PACE | HR | REST HR | RUN TYPE | SHOES | NOTES |
|------|----------|------|------|----|---------|----------|-------|-------|
|      |          |      |      |    |         |          |       |       |

| DATE | DISTANCE | TIME | PACE | HR | REST HR | RUN TYPE | SHOES | NOTES |
|------|----------|------|------|----|---------|----------|-------|-------|
|      |          |      |      |    |         |          |       |       |

# RUNNING / JOGGING LOG

YEAR          MONTH

| DATE | DISTANCE | TIME | PACE | HR | REST HR | RUN TYPE | SHOES | NOTES |
|------|----------|------|------|----|---------|----------|-------|-------|
|      |          |      |      |    |         |          |       |       |

| DATE | DISTANCE | TIME | PACE | HR | REST HR | RUN TYPE | SHOES | NOTES |
|------|----------|------|------|----|---------|----------|-------|-------|

# RUNNING / JOGGING LOG

YEAR          MONTH

| DATE | DISTANCE | TIME | PACE | HR | REST HR | RUN TYPE | SHOES | NOTES |
|------|----------|------|------|-----|---------|----------|-------|-------|
|      |          |      |      |     |         |          |       |       |
|      |          |      |      |     |         |          |       |       |
|      |          |      |      |     |         |          |       |       |
|      |          |      |      |     |         |          |       |       |
|      |          |      |      |     |         |          |       |       |
|      |          |      |      |     |         |          |       |       |
|      |          |      |      |     |         |          |       |       |
|      |          |      |      |     |         |          |       |       |
|      |          |      |      |     |         |          |       |       |
|      |          |      |      |     |         |          |       |       |
|      |          |      |      |     |         |          |       |       |
|      |          |      |      |     |         |          |       |       |
|      |          |      |      |     |         |          |       |       |
|      |          |      |      |     |         |          |       |       |
|      |          |      |      |     |         |          |       |       |
|      |          |      |      |     |         |          |       |       |
| DATE | DISTANCE | TIME | PACE | HR | REST HR | RUN TYPE | SHOES | NOTES |
|      |          |      |      |     |         |          |       |       |

# RUNNING / JOGGING LOG

YEAR          MONTH

| DATE | DISTANCE | TIME | PACE | HR | REST HR | RUN TYPE | SHOES | NOTES |
|------|----------|------|------|----|---------|----------|-------|-------|
| | | | | | | | | |
| | | | | | | | | |
| | | | | | | | | |
| | | | | | | | | |
| | | | | | | | | |
| | | | | | | | | |
| | | | | | | | | |
| | | | | | | | | |
| | | | | | | | | |
| | | | | | | | | |
| | | | | | | | | |
| | | | | | | | | |
| | | | | | | | | |
| | | | | | | | | |
| | | | | | | | | |
| | | | | | | | | |
| | | | | | | | | |
| | | | | | | | | |
| | | | | | | | | |
| | | | | | | | | |

| DATE | DISTANCE | TIME | PACE | HR | REST HR | RUN TYPE | SHOES | NOTES |
|------|----------|------|------|----|---------|----------|-------|-------|

# RUNNING / JOGGING LOG

YEAR       MONTH

| DATE | DISTANCE | TIME | PACE | HR | REST HR | RUN TYPE | SHOES | NOTES |
|------|----------|------|------|----|---------|----------|-------|-------|
|      |          |      |      |    |         |          |       |       |

| DATE | DISTANCE | TIME | PACE | HR | REST HR | RUN TYPE | SHOES | NOTES |
|------|----------|------|------|----|---------|----------|-------|-------|
|      |          |      |      |    |         |          |       |       |

# RUNNING / JOGGING LOG

YEAR __________ MONTH __________

| DATE | DISTANCE | TIME | PACE | HR | REST HR | RUN TYPE | SHOES | | NOTES |
|------|----------|------|------|----|---------|----------|-------|--|-------|
|      |          |      |      |    |         |          |       |  |       |
|      |          |      |      |    |         |          |       |  |       |
|      |          |      |      |    |         |          |       |  |       |
|      |          |      |      |    |         |          |       |  |       |
|      |          |      |      |    |         |          |       |  |       |
|      |          |      |      |    |         |          |       |  |       |
|      |          |      |      |    |         |          |       |  |       |
|      |          |      |      |    |         |          |       |  |       |
|      |          |      |      |    |         |          |       |  |       |
|      |          |      |      |    |         |          |       |  |       |
|      |          |      |      |    |         |          |       |  |       |
|      |          |      |      |    |         |          |       |  |       |
|      |          |      |      |    |         |          |       |  |       |
|      |          |      |      |    |         |          |       |  |       |
|      |          |      |      |    |         |          |       |  |       |
|      |          |      |      |    |         |          |       |  |       |
| DATE | DISTANCE | TIME | PACE | HR | REST HR | RUN TYPE | SHOES | | NOTES |
|      |          |      |      |    |         |          |       |  |       |

# RUNNING / JOGGING LOG

YEAR           MONTH

| DATE | DISTANCE | TIME | PACE | HR | REST HR | RUN TYPE | SHOES | NOTES |
|------|----------|------|------|-----|---------|----------|-------|-------|
|      |          |      |      |     |         |          |       |       |

| DATE | DISTANCE | TIME | PACE | HR | REST HR | RUN TYPE | SHOES | NOTES |
|------|----------|------|------|-----|---------|----------|-------|-------|
|      |          |      |      |     |         |          |       |       |

# RUNNING / JOGGING LOG

YEAR ________   MONTH ________

| DATE | DISTANCE | TIME | PACE | HR | REST HR | RUN TYPE | SHOES | NOTES |
|------|----------|------|------|-----|---------|----------|-------|-------|
|  |  |  |  |  |  |  |  |  |
|  |  |  |  |  |  |  |  |  |
|  |  |  |  |  |  |  |  |  |
|  |  |  |  |  |  |  |  |  |
|  |  |  |  |  |  |  |  |  |
|  |  |  |  |  |  |  |  |  |
|  |  |  |  |  |  |  |  |  |
|  |  |  |  |  |  |  |  |  |
|  |  |  |  |  |  |  |  |  |
|  |  |  |  |  |  |  |  |  |
|  |  |  |  |  |  |  |  |  |
|  |  |  |  |  |  |  |  |  |
|  |  |  |  |  |  |  |  |  |
|  |  |  |  |  |  |  |  |  |
|  |  |  |  |  |  |  |  |  |
|  |  |  |  |  |  |  |  |  |
|  |  |  |  |  |  |  |  |  |
|  |  |  |  |  |  |  |  |  |

# RUNNING / JOGGING LOG

YEAR ____________ MONTH ____________

| DATE | DISTANCE | TIME | PACE | HR | REST HR | RUN TYPE | SHOES | | NOTES |
|------|----------|------|------|-----|---------|----------|-------|--|-------|
|  |  |  |  |  |  |  |  |  |  |
|  |  |  |  |  |  |  |  |  |  |
|  |  |  |  |  |  |  |  |  |  |
|  |  |  |  |  |  |  |  |  |  |
|  |  |  |  |  |  |  |  |  |  |
|  |  |  |  |  |  |  |  |  |  |
|  |  |  |  |  |  |  |  |  |  |
|  |  |  |  |  |  |  |  |  |  |
|  |  |  |  |  |  |  |  |  |  |
|  |  |  |  |  |  |  |  |  |  |
|  |  |  |  |  |  |  |  |  |  |
|  |  |  |  |  |  |  |  |  |  |
|  |  |  |  |  |  |  |  |  |  |
|  |  |  |  |  |  |  |  |  |  |
|  |  |  |  |  |  |  |  |  |  |
| DATE | DISTANCE | TIME | PACE | HR | REST HR | RUN TYPE | SHOES | | NOTES |

# RUNNING / JOGGING LOG

YEAR _______  MONTH _______

| DATE | DISTANCE | TIME | PACE | HR | REST HR | RUN TYPE | SHOES | | NOTES |
|------|----------|------|------|-----|---------|----------|-------|--|-------|
|      |          |      |      |     |         |          |       |  |       |
|      |          |      |      |     |         |          |       |  |       |
|      |          |      |      |     |         |          |       |  |       |
|      |          |      |      |     |         |          |       |  |       |
|      |          |      |      |     |         |          |       |  |       |
|      |          |      |      |     |         |          |       |  |       |
|      |          |      |      |     |         |          |       |  |       |
|      |          |      |      |     |         |          |       |  |       |
|      |          |      |      |     |         |          |       |  |       |
|      |          |      |      |     |         |          |       |  |       |
|      |          |      |      |     |         |          |       |  |       |
|      |          |      |      |     |         |          |       |  |       |
|      |          |      |      |     |         |          |       |  |       |
|      |          |      |      |     |         |          |       |  |       |
|      |          |      |      |     |         |          |       |  |       |
|      |          |      |      |     |         |          |       |  |       |
|      |          |      |      |     |         |          |       |  |       |
|      |          |      |      |     |         |          |       |  |       |

| DATE | DISTANCE | TIME | PACE | HR | REST HR | RUN TYPE | SHOES | | NOTES |
|------|----------|------|------|-----|---------|----------|-------|--|-------|

# RUNNING / JOGGING LOG

YEAR      MONTH

| DATE | DISTANCE | TIME | PACE | HR | REST HR | RUN TYPE | SHOES | NOTES |
|------|----------|------|------|-----|---------|----------|-------|-------|
|  |  |  |  |  |  |  |  |  |
|  |  |  |  |  |  |  |  |  |
|  |  |  |  |  |  |  |  |  |
|  |  |  |  |  |  |  |  |  |
|  |  |  |  |  |  |  |  |  |
|  |  |  |  |  |  |  |  |  |
|  |  |  |  |  |  |  |  |  |

| DATE | DISTANCE | TIME | PACE | HR | REST HR | RUN TYPE | SHOES | NOTES |
|------|----------|------|------|-----|---------|----------|-------|-------|

# RUNNING / JOGGING LOG

YEAR          MONTH

| DATE | DISTANCE | TIME | PACE | HR | REST HR | RUN TYPE | SHOES | NOTES |
|------|----------|------|------|-----|---------|----------|-------|-------|
|      |          |      |      |     |         |          |       |       |
|      |          |      |      |     |         |          |       |       |
|      |          |      |      |     |         |          |       |       |
|      |          |      |      |     |         |          |       |       |
|      |          |      |      |     |         |          |       |       |
|      |          |      |      |     |         |          |       |       |
|      |          |      |      |     |         |          |       |       |
|      |          |      |      |     |         |          |       |       |
|      |          |      |      |     |         |          |       |       |
|      |          |      |      |     |         |          |       |       |
|      |          |      |      |     |         |          |       |       |
|      |          |      |      |     |         |          |       |       |
|      |          |      |      |     |         |          |       |       |
|      |          |      |      |     |         |          |       |       |
|      |          |      |      |     |         |          |       |       |
|      |          |      |      |     |         |          |       |       |
|      |          |      |      |     |         |          |       |       |
|      |          |      |      |     |         |          |       |       |
|      |          |      |      |     |         |          |       |       |
|      |          |      |      |     |         |          |       |       |

| DATE | DISTANCE | TIME | PACE | HR | REST HR | RUN TYPE | SHOES | NOTES |
|------|----------|------|------|-----|---------|----------|-------|-------|

# RUNNING / JOGGING LOG

YEAR      MONTH

| DATE | DISTANCE | TIME | PACE | HR | REST HR | RUN TYPE | SHOES | NOTES |
|------|----------|------|------|-----|---------|----------|-------|-------|
|  |  |  |  |  |  |  |  |  |
|  |  |  |  |  |  |  |  |  |
|  |  |  |  |  |  |  |  |  |
|  |  |  |  |  |  |  |  |  |
|  |  |  |  |  |  |  |  |  |
|  |  |  |  |  |  |  |  |  |
|  |  |  |  |  |  |  |  |  |
|  |  |  |  |  |  |  |  |  |
|  |  |  |  |  |  |  |  |  |
|  |  |  |  |  |  |  |  |  |
|  |  |  |  |  |  |  |  |  |
|  |  |  |  |  |  |  |  |  |
|  |  |  |  |  |  |  |  |  |
|  |  |  |  |  |  |  |  |  |
|  |  |  |  |  |  |  |  |  |
|  |  |  |  |  |  |  |  |  |
| DATE | DISTANCE | TIME | PACE | HR | REST HR | RUN TYPE | SHOES | NOTES |
|  |  |  |  |  |  |  |  |  |

# RUNNING / JOGGING LOG

YEAR      MONTH

| DATE | DISTANCE | TIME | PACE | HR | REST HR | RUN TYPE | SHOES | NOTES |
|------|----------|------|------|----|---------|----------|-------|-------|
| | | | | | | | | |
| | | | | | | | | |
| | | | | | | | | |
| | | | | | | | | |
| | | | | | | | | |
| | | | | | | | | |
| | | | | | | | | |
| | | | | | | | | |
| | | | | | | | | |
| | | | | | | | | |
| | | | | | | | | |
| | | | | | | | | |
| | | | | | | | | |
| | | | | | | | | |
| | | | | | | | | |
| | | | | | | | | |

# RUNNING / JOGGING LOG

YEAR            MONTH

| DATE | DISTANCE | TIME | PACE | HR | REST HR | RUN TYPE | SHOES | NOTES |
|------|----------|------|------|----|---------|----------|-------|-------|
|      |          |      |      |    |         |          |       |       |
|      |          |      |      |    |         |          |       |       |
|      |          |      |      |    |         |          |       |       |
|      |          |      |      |    |         |          |       |       |
|      |          |      |      |    |         |          |       |       |
|      |          |      |      |    |         |          |       |       |
|      |          |      |      |    |         |          |       |       |
|      |          |      |      |    |         |          |       |       |
|      |          |      |      |    |         |          |       |       |
|      |          |      |      |    |         |          |       |       |
|      |          |      |      |    |         |          |       |       |
|      |          |      |      |    |         |          |       |       |
|      |          |      |      |    |         |          |       |       |
|      |          |      |      |    |         |          |       |       |
|      |          |      |      |    |         |          |       |       |
|      |          |      |      |    |         |          |       |       |
|      |          |      |      |    |         |          |       |       |
| DATE | DISTANCE | TIME | PACE | HR | REST HR | RUN TYPE | SHOES | NOTES |

# RUNNING / JOGGING LOG

YEAR          MONTH

| DATE | DISTANCE | TIME | PACE | HR | REST HR | RUN TYPE | SHOES | NOTES |
|------|----------|------|------|----|---------|----------|-------|-------|
|      |          |      |      |    |         |          |       |       |
|      |          |      |      |    |         |          |       |       |
|      |          |      |      |    |         |          |       |       |
|      |          |      |      |    |         |          |       |       |
|      |          |      |      |    |         |          |       |       |
|      |          |      |      |    |         |          |       |       |
|      |          |      |      |    |         |          |       |       |
|      |          |      |      |    |         |          |       |       |
|      |          |      |      |    |         |          |       |       |
|      |          |      |      |    |         |          |       |       |

| DATE | DISTANCE | TIME | PACE | HR | REST HR | RUN TYPE | SHOES | NOTES |
|------|----------|------|------|----|---------|----------|-------|-------|
|      |          |      |      |    |         |          |       |       |

# RUNNING / JOGGING LOG

YEAR       MONTH

| DATE | DISTANCE | TIME | PACE | HR | REST HR | RUN TYPE | SHOES | NOTES |
|------|----------|------|------|----|---------|----------|-------|-------|
|      |          |      |      |    |         |          |       |       |

| DATE | DISTANCE | TIME | PACE | HR | REST HR | RUN TYPE | SHOES | NOTES |
|------|----------|------|------|----|---------|----------|-------|-------|
|      |          |      |      |    |         |          |       |       |

# RUNNING / JOGGING LOG

YEAR _______ MONTH _______

| DATE | DISTANCE | TIME | PACE | HR | REST HR | RUN TYPE | SHOES | NOTES |
|---|---|---|---|---|---|---|---|---|
| | | | | | | | | |
| | | | | | | | | |
| | | | | | | | | |
| | | | | | | | | |
| | | | | | | | | |
| | | | | | | | | |
| | | | | | | | | |
| | | | | | | | | |
| | | | | | | | | |
| | | | | | | | | |
| | | | | | | | | |
| | | | | | | | | |
| | | | | | | | | |
| | | | | | | | | |
| | | | | | | | | |
| | | | | | | | | |
| | | | | | | | | |
| | | | | | | | | |
| | | | | | | | | |
| | | | | | | | | |
| DATE | DISTANCE | TIME | PACE | HR | REST HR | RUN TYPE | SHOES | NOTES |

# RUNNING / JOGGING LOG

YEAR _______    MONTH _______

| DATE | DISTANCE | TIME | PACE | HR | REST HR | RUN TYPE | SHOES | NOTES |
|------|----------|------|------|----|---------|----------|-------|-------|
|      |          |      |      |    |         |          |       |       |
|      |          |      |      |    |         |          |       |       |
|      |          |      |      |    |         |          |       |       |
|      |          |      |      |    |         |          |       |       |
|      |          |      |      |    |         |          |       |       |
|      |          |      |      |    |         |          |       |       |
|      |          |      |      |    |         |          |       |       |
|      |          |      |      |    |         |          |       |       |
|      |          |      |      |    |         |          |       |       |
|      |          |      |      |    |         |          |       |       |
|      |          |      |      |    |         |          |       |       |
|      |          |      |      |    |         |          |       |       |
| DATE | DISTANCE | TIME | PACE | HR | REST HR | RUN TYPE | SHOES | NOTES |

# RUNNING / JOGGING LOG

YEAR ______  MONTH ______

| DATE | DISTANCE | TIME | PACE | HR | REST HR | RUN TYPE | SHOES | NOTES |
|------|----------|------|------|----|---------|----------|-------|-------|
|      |          |      |      |    |         |          |       |       |

# RUNNING / JOGGING LOG

YEAR ________  MONTH ________

| DATE | DISTANCE | TIME | PACE | HR | REST HR | RUN TYPE | SHOES | NOTES |
|------|----------|------|------|----|---------|----------|-------|-------|
|  |  |  |  |  |  |  |  |  |

| DATE | DISTANCE | TIME | PACE | HR | REST HR | RUN TYPE | SHOES | NOTES |
|------|----------|------|------|----|---------|----------|-------|-------|
|  |  |  |  |  |  |  |  |  |

# RUNNING / JOGGING LOG

YEAR          MONTH

| DATE | DISTANCE | TIME | PACE | HR | REST HR | RUN TYPE | SHOES | NOTES |
|---|---|---|---|---|---|---|---|---|
| | | | | | | | | |
| | | | | | | | | |
| | | | | | | | | |
| | | | | | | | | |
| | | | | | | | | |
| | | | | | | | | |
| | | | | | | | | |
| | | | | | | | | |
| | | | | | | | | |
| | | | | | | | | |
| | | | | | | | | |
| | | | | | | | | |
| | | | | | | | | |
| | | | | | | | | |
| | | | | | | | | |
| | | | | | | | | |
| | | | | | | | | |
| | | | | | | | | |
| | | | | | | | | |

| DATE | DISTANCE | TIME | PACE | HR | REST HR | RUN TYPE | SHOES | NOTES |
|---|---|---|---|---|---|---|---|---|
| | | | | | | | | |

# RUNNING / JOGGING LOG

YEAR _______ MONTH _______

| DATE | DISTANCE | TIME | PACE | HR | REST HR | RUN TYPE | SHOES | NOTES |
|------|----------|------|------|----|---------|----------|-------|-------|
| | | | | | | | | |
| | | | | | | | | |
| | | | | | | | | |
| | | | | | | | | |
| | | | | | | | | |
| | | | | | | | | |
| | | | | | | | | |
| | | | | | | | | |
| | | | | | | | | |
| | | | | | | | | |
| | | | | | | | | |
| | | | | | | | | |
| | | | | | | | | |
| | | | | | | | | |
| | | | | | | | | |
| | | | | | | | | |
| | | | | | | | | |
| DATE | DISTANCE | TIME | PACE | HR | REST HR | RUN TYPE | SHOES | NOTES |
| | | | | | | | | |

# RUNNING / JOGGING LOG

YEAR                MONTH

| DATE | DISTANCE | TIME | PACE | HR | REST HR | RUN TYPE | SHOES | NOTES |
|------|----------|------|------|-----|---------|----------|-------|-------|
|      |          |      |      |     |         |          |       |       |
|      |          |      |      |     |         |          |       |       |
|      |          |      |      |     |         |          |       |       |
|      |          |      |      |     |         |          |       |       |
|      |          |      |      |     |         |          |       |       |
|      |          |      |      |     |         |          |       |       |
|      |          |      |      |     |         |          |       |       |
|      |          |      |      |     |         |          |       |       |
|      |          |      |      |     |         |          |       |       |
|      |          |      |      |     |         |          |       |       |
|      |          |      |      |     |         |          |       |       |
|      |          |      |      |     |         |          |       |       |
|      |          |      |      |     |         |          |       |       |
|      |          |      |      |     |         |          |       |       |
|      |          |      |      |     |         |          |       |       |
|      |          |      |      |     |         |          |       |       |

# RUNNING / JOGGING LOG

YEAR ________  MONTH ________

| DATE | DISTANCE | TIME | PACE | HR | REST HR | RUN TYPE | SHOES | NOTES |
|------|----------|------|------|----|---------|----------|-------|-------|
|      |          |      |      |    |         |          |       |       |
|      |          |      |      |    |         |          |       |       |
|      |          |      |      |    |         |          |       |       |

| DATE | DISTANCE | TIME | PACE | HR | REST HR | RUN TYPE | SHOES | NOTES |
|------|----------|------|------|----|---------|----------|-------|-------|
|      |          |      |      |    |         |          |       |       |

# RUNNING / JOGGING LOG

YEAR  MONTH

| DATE | DISTANCE | TIME | PACE | HR | REST HR | RUN TYPE | SHOES | | NOTES |
|------|----------|------|------|----|---------|----------|-------|--|-------|
| | | | | | | | | | |
| | | | | | | | | | |
| | | | | | | | | | |
| | | | | | | | | | |
| | | | | | | | | | |
| | | | | | | | | | |
| | | | | | | | | | |
| | | | | | | | | | |
| | | | | | | | | | |
| | | | | | | | | | |
| | | | | | | | | | |
| | | | | | | | | | |
| | | | | | | | | | |
| | | | | | | | | | |
| | | | | | | | | | |

# RUNNING / JOGGING LOG

YEAR      MONTH

| DATE | DISTANCE | TIME | PACE | HR | REST HR | RUN TYPE | SHOES | NOTES |
|------|----------|------|------|----|---------|----------|-------|-------|
|      |          |      |      |    |         |          |       |       |
|      |          |      |      |    |         |          |       |       |
|      |          |      |      |    |         |          |       |       |
|      |          |      |      |    |         |          |       |       |
|      |          |      |      |    |         |          |       |       |
|      |          |      |      |    |         |          |       |       |
|      |          |      |      |    |         |          |       |       |
|      |          |      |      |    |         |          |       |       |
|      |          |      |      |    |         |          |       |       |
|      |          |      |      |    |         |          |       |       |
|      |          |      |      |    |         |          |       |       |
|      |          |      |      |    |         |          |       |       |
|      |          |      |      |    |         |          |       |       |
|      |          |      |      |    |         |          |       |       |
|      |          |      |      |    |         |          |       |       |
| DATE | DISTANCE | TIME | PACE | HR | REST HR | RUN TYPE | SHOES | NOTES |
|      |          |      |      |    |         |          |       |       |

# RUNNING / JOGGING LOG

YEAR ________    MONTH ________

| DATE | DISTANCE | TIME | PACE | HR | REST HR | RUN TYPE | SHOES | NOTES |
|------|----------|------|------|----|---------|----------|-------|-------|
|      |          |      |      |    |         |          |       |       |
|      |          |      |      |    |         |          |       |       |
|      |          |      |      |    |         |          |       |       |
|      |          |      |      |    |         |          |       |       |
|      |          |      |      |    |         |          |       |       |
|      |          |      |      |    |         |          |       |       |
|      |          |      |      |    |         |          |       |       |
|      |          |      |      |    |         |          |       |       |
|      |          |      |      |    |         |          |       |       |
|      |          |      |      |    |         |          |       |       |
| DATE | DISTANCE | TIME | PACE | HR | REST HR | RUN TYPE | SHOES | NOTES |

# RUNNING / JOGGING LOG

YEAR            MONTH

| DATE | DISTANCE | TIME | PACE | HR | REST HR | RUN TYPE | SHOES | NOTES |
|------|----------|------|------|----|---------|----------|-------|-------|
|      |          |      |      |    |         |          |       |       |
|      |          |      |      |    |         |          |       |       |
|      |          |      |      |    |         |          |       |       |
|      |          |      |      |    |         |          |       |       |
|      |          |      |      |    |         |          |       |       |
|      |          |      |      |    |         |          |       |       |
|      |          |      |      |    |         |          |       |       |
|      |          |      |      |    |         |          |       |       |
|      |          |      |      |    |         |          |       |       |
|      |          |      |      |    |         |          |       |       |

| DATE | DISTANCE | TIME | PACE | HR | REST HR | RUN TYPE | SHOES | NOTES |
|------|----------|------|------|----|---------|----------|-------|-------|

# RUNNING / JOGGING LOG

YEAR       MONTH

| DATE | DISTANCE | TIME | PACE | HR | REST HR | RUN TYPE | SHOES | NOTES |
|------|----------|------|------|-----|---------|----------|-------|-------|
|      |          |      |      |     |         |          |       |       |
|      |          |      |      |     |         |          |       |       |
|      |          |      |      |     |         |          |       |       |
|      |          |      |      |     |         |          |       |       |
|      |          |      |      |     |         |          |       |       |
|      |          |      |      |     |         |          |       |       |
|      |          |      |      |     |         |          |       |       |
|      |          |      |      |     |         |          |       |       |
|      |          |      |      |     |         |          |       |       |
|      |          |      |      |     |         |          |       |       |
| DATE | DISTANCE | TIME | PACE | HR | REST HR | RUN TYPE | SHOES | NOTES |

# RUNNING / JOGGING LOG

YEAR _______ MONTH _______

| DATE | DISTANCE | TIME | PACE | HR | REST HR | RUN TYPE | SHOES | NOTES |
|------|----------|------|------|-----|---------|----------|-------|-------|
|      |          |      |      |     |         |          |       |       |
|      |          |      |      |     |         |          |       |       |
|      |          |      |      |     |         |          |       |       |
|      |          |      |      |     |         |          |       |       |
|      |          |      |      |     |         |          |       |       |
|      |          |      |      |     |         |          |       |       |
|      |          |      |      |     |         |          |       |       |
|      |          |      |      |     |         |          |       |       |
|      |          |      |      |     |         |          |       |       |
|      |          |      |      |     |         |          |       |       |
|      |          |      |      |     |         |          |       |       |
|      |          |      |      |     |         |          |       |       |
|      |          |      |      |     |         |          |       |       |
|      |          |      |      |     |         |          |       |       |
|      |          |      |      |     |         |          |       |       |
|      |          |      |      |     |         |          |       |       |
|      |          |      |      |     |         |          |       |       |
|      |          |      |      |     |         |          |       |       |
|      |          |      |      |     |         |          |       |       |
| DATE | DISTANCE | TIME | PACE | HR | REST HR | RUN TYPE | SHOES | NOTES |

# RUNNING / JOGGING LOG

YEAR      MONTH

| DATE | DISTANCE | TIME | PACE | HR | REST HR | RUN TYPE | SHOES | | NOTES |
|------|----------|------|------|----|---------|----------|-------|---|-------|
| | | | | | | | | | |
| | | | | | | | | | |
| | | | | | | | | | |
| | | | | | | | | | |
| | | | | | | | | | |
| | | | | | | | | | |
| | | | | | | | | | |
| | | | | | | | | | |
| | | | | | | | | | |
| | | | | | | | | | |
| | | | | | | | | | |
| | | | | | | | | | |
| | | | | | | | | | |
| | | | | | | | | | |
| | | | | | | | | | |
| | | | | | | | | | |
| | | | | | | | | | |
| | | | | | | | | | |
| | | | | | | | | | |
| | | | | | | | | | |
| | | | | | | | | | |
| | | | | | | | | | |

# RUNNING / JOGGING LOG

YEAR       MONTH

| DATE | DISTANCE | TIME | PACE | HR | REST HR | RUN TYPE | SHOES | NOTES |
|------|----------|------|------|-----|---------|----------|-------|-------|
|  |  |  |  |  |  |  |  |  |
|  |  |  |  |  |  |  |  |  |
|  |  |  |  |  |  |  |  |  |
|  |  |  |  |  |  |  |  |  |
|  |  |  |  |  |  |  |  |  |
|  |  |  |  |  |  |  |  |  |
|  |  |  |  |  |  |  |  |  |
|  |  |  |  |  |  |  |  |  |
|  |  |  |  |  |  |  |  |  |
|  |  |  |  |  |  |  |  |  |

| DATE | DISTANCE | TIME | PACE | HR | REST HR | RUN TYPE | SHOES | NOTES |
|------|----------|------|------|-----|---------|----------|-------|-------|
|  |  |  |  |  |  |  |  |  |
|  |  |  |  |  |  |  |  |  |
|  |  |  |  |  |  |  |  |  |

# RUNNING / JOGGING LOG

YEAR      MONTH

| DATE | DISTANCE | TIME | PACE | HR | REST HR | RUN TYPE | SHOES | | NOTES |
|------|----------|------|------|----|---------|----------|-------|--|-------|
| | | | | | | | | | |

# RUNNING / JOGGING LOG

YEAR            MONTH

| DATE | DISTANCE | TIME | PACE | HR | REST HR | RUN TYPE | SHOES | NOTES |
|------|----------|------|------|----|---------|----------|-------|-------|
|      |          |      |      |    |         |          |       |       |

| DATE | DISTANCE | TIME | PACE | HR | REST HR | RUN TYPE | SHOES | NOTES |
|------|----------|------|------|----|---------|----------|-------|-------|

# RUNNING / JOGGING LOG

YEAR　　　　MONTH

| DATE | DISTANCE | TIME | PACE | HR | REST HR | RUN TYPE | SHOES | | NOTES |
|------|----------|------|------|----|---------|----------|-------|---|-------|
| | | | | | | | | | |
| | | | | | | | | | |
| | | | | | | | | | |
| | | | | | | | | | |
| | | | | | | | | | |
| | | | | | | | | | |
| | | | | | | | | | |
| | | | | | | | | | |
| | | | | | | | | | |
| | | | | | | | | | |
| | | | | | | | | | |
| | | | | | | | | | |
| | | | | | | | | | |
| | | | | | | | | | |
| | | | | | | | | | |
| | | | | | | | | | |
| | | | | | | | | | |

| DATE | DISTANCE | TIME | PACE | HR | REST HR | RUN TYPE | SHOES | | NOTES |
|------|----------|------|------|----|---------|----------|-------|---|-------|
| | | | | | | | | | |
| | | | | | | | | | |

# RUNNING / JOGGING LOG

YEAR      MONTH

| DATE | DISTANCE | TIME | PACE | HR | REST HR | RUN TYPE | SHOES | | NOTES |
|------|----------|------|------|----|---------|----------|-------|--|-------|
| | | | | | | | | | |
| | | | | | | | | | |
| | | | | | | | | | |
| | | | | | | | | | |
| | | | | | | | | | |
| | | | | | | | | | |
| | | | | | | | | | |
| DATE | DISTANCE | TIME | PACE | HR | REST HR | RUN TYPE | SHOES | | NOTES |

# RUNNING / JOGGING LOG

YEAR       MONTH

| DATE | DISTANCE | TIME | PACE | HR | REST HR | RUN TYPE | SHOES | NOTES |
|------|----------|------|------|----|---------|----------|-------|-------|
|  |  |  |  |  |  |  |  |  |
|  |  |  |  |  |  |  |  |  |
|  |  |  |  |  |  |  |  |  |
|  |  |  |  |  |  |  |  |  |
|  |  |  |  |  |  |  |  |  |
|  |  |  |  |  |  |  |  |  |
|  |  |  |  |  |  |  |  |  |
|  |  |  |  |  |  |  |  |  |
|  |  |  |  |  |  |  |  |  |
|  |  |  |  |  |  |  |  |  |
|  |  |  |  |  |  |  |  |  |
|  |  |  |  |  |  |  |  |  |
|  |  |  |  |  |  |  |  |  |
|  |  |  |  |  |  |  |  |  |
|  |  |  |  |  |  |  |  |  |
|  |  |  |  |  |  |  |  |  |

| DATE | DISTANCE | TIME | PACE | HR | REST HR | RUN TYPE | SHOES | NOTES |
|------|----------|------|------|----|---------|----------|-------|-------|
|  |  |  |  |  |  |  |  |  |
|  |  |  |  |  |  |  |  |  |

# RUNNING / JOGGING LOG

YEAR _______ MONTH _______

| DATE | DISTANCE | TIME | PACE | HR | REST HR | RUN TYPE | SHOES | NOTES |
|------|----------|------|------|----|---------|----------|-------|-------|
|      |          |      |      |    |         |          |       |       |
|      |          |      |      |    |         |          |       |       |
|      |          |      |      |    |         |          |       |       |
|      |          |      |      |    |         |          |       |       |
|      |          |      |      |    |         |          |       |       |
|      |          |      |      |    |         |          |       |       |
|      |          |      |      |    |         |          |       |       |
|      |          |      |      |    |         |          |       |       |
|      |          |      |      |    |         |          |       |       |
|      |          |      |      |    |         |          |       |       |
|      |          |      |      |    |         |          |       |       |
|      |          |      |      |    |         |          |       |       |
|      |          |      |      |    |         |          |       |       |
|      |          |      |      |    |         |          |       |       |
|      |          |      |      |    |         |          |       |       |

| DATE | DISTANCE | TIME | PACE | HR | REST HR | RUN TYPE | SHOES | NOTES |
|------|----------|------|------|----|---------|----------|-------|-------|
|      |          |      |      |    |         |          |       |       |
|      |          |      |      |    |         |          |       |       |

# RUNNING / JOGGING LOG

YEAR __________  MONTH __________

| DATE | DISTANCE | TIME | PACE | HR | REST HR | RUN TYPE | SHOES | NOTES |
|------|----------|------|------|----|---------|----------|-------|-------|
|      |          |      |      |    |         |          |       |       |

# RUNNING / JOGGING LOG

YEAR　　　　MONTH

| DATE | DISTANCE | TIME | PACE | HR | REST HR | RUN TYPE | SHOES | NOTES |
|------|----------|------|------|----|---------|----------|-------|-------|
|      |          |      |      |    |         |          |       |       |
|      |          |      |      |    |         |          |       |       |
|      |          |      |      |    |         |          |       |       |
|      |          |      |      |    |         |          |       |       |
|      |          |      |      |    |         |          |       |       |
|      |          |      |      |    |         |          |       |       |
|      |          |      |      |    |         |          |       |       |
|      |          |      |      |    |         |          |       |       |
|      |          |      |      |    |         |          |       |       |
|      |          |      |      |    |         |          |       |       |
|      |          |      |      |    |         |          |       |       |
|      |          |      |      |    |         |          |       |       |
|      |          |      |      |    |         |          |       |       |
|      |          |      |      |    |         |          |       |       |
|      |          |      |      |    |         |          |       |       |
|      |          |      |      |    |         |          |       |       |
|      |          |      |      |    |         |          |       |       |
|      |          |      |      |    |         |          |       |       |
| DATE | DISTANCE | TIME | PACE | HR | REST HR | RUN TYPE | SHOES | NOTES |

# RUNNING / JOGGING LOG

YEAR ............... MONTH ...............

| DATE | DISTANCE | TIME | PACE | HR | REST HR | RUN TYPE | SHOES | | NOTES |
|------|----------|------|------|-----|---------|----------|-------|---|-------|
| | | | | | | | | | |

# RUNNING / JOGGING LOG

YEAR ............ MONTH ............

| DATE | DISTANCE | TIME | PACE | HR | REST HR | RUN TYPE | SHOES | | NOTES |
|------|----------|------|------|----|---------|----------|-------|--|-------|
| | | | | | | | | | |

| DATE | DISTANCE | TIME | PACE | HR | REST HR | RUN TYPE | SHOES | | NOTES |
|------|----------|------|------|----|---------|----------|-------|--|-------|
| | | | | | | | | | |

# RUNNING / JOGGING LOG

YEAR ________  MONTH ________

| DATE | DISTANCE | TIME | PACE | HR | REST HR | RUN TYPE | SHOES | NOTES |
|------|----------|------|------|----|---------|----------|-------|-------|
|      |          |      |      |    |         |          |       |       |
|      |          |      |      |    |         |          |       |       |
|      |          |      |      |    |         |          |       |       |
|      |          |      |      |    |         |          |       |       |
|      |          |      |      |    |         |          |       |       |
|      |          |      |      |    |         |          |       |       |
|      |          |      |      |    |         |          |       |       |
|      |          |      |      |    |         |          |       |       |
|      |          |      |      |    |         |          |       |       |
|      |          |      |      |    |         |          |       |       |
|      |          |      |      |    |         |          |       |       |
|      |          |      |      |    |         |          |       |       |

YEAR ________  MONTH ________

| DATE | DISTANCE | TIME | PACE | HR | REST HR | RUN TYPE | SHOES | NOTES |
|------|----------|------|------|----|---------|----------|-------|-------|
|      |          |      |      |    |         |          |       |       |
|      |          |      |      |    |         |          |       |       |

# RUNNING / JOGGING LOG

YEAR ____________  MONTH ____________

| DATE | DISTANCE | TIME | PACE | HR | REST HR | RUN TYPE | SHOES | NOTES |
|------|----------|------|------|----|---------|----------|-------|-------|
|  |  |  |  |  |  |  |  |  |
|  |  |  |  |  |  |  |  |  |
|  |  |  |  |  |  |  |  |  |
|  |  |  |  |  |  |  |  |  |
|  |  |  |  |  |  |  |  |  |
|  |  |  |  |  |  |  |  |  |
|  |  |  |  |  |  |  |  |  |
|  |  |  |  |  |  |  |  |  |
|  |  |  |  |  |  |  |  |  |
|  |  |  |  |  |  |  |  |  |
|  |  |  |  |  |  |  |  |  |
|  |  |  |  |  |  |  |  |  |
|  |  |  |  |  |  |  |  |  |

| DATE | DISTANCE | TIME | PACE | HR | REST HR | RUN TYPE | SHOES | NOTES |
|------|----------|------|------|----|---------|----------|-------|-------|
|  |  |  |  |  |  |  |  |  |
|  |  |  |  |  |  |  |  |  |

# RUNNING / JOGGING LOG

YEAR      MONTH

| DATE | DISTANCE | TIME | PACE | HR | REST HR | RUN TYPE | SHOES | | NOTES |
|------|----------|------|------|----|---------|----------|-------|---|-------|
|  |  |  |  |  |  |  |  |  |  |

# RUNNING / JOGGING LOG

YEAR ________  MONTH ________

| DATE | DISTANCE | TIME | PACE | HR | REST HR | RUN TYPE | SHOES | NOTES |
|------|----------|------|------|-----|---------|----------|-------|-------|
|  |  |  |  |  |  |  |  |  |
|  |  |  |  |  |  |  |  |  |
|  |  |  |  |  |  |  |  |  |
|  |  |  |  |  |  |  |  |  |
|  |  |  |  |  |  |  |  |  |
|  |  |  |  |  |  |  |  |  |
|  |  |  |  |  |  |  |  |  |
|  |  |  |  |  |  |  |  |  |
|  |  |  |  |  |  |  |  |  |
|  |  |  |  |  |  |  |  |  |
|  |  |  |  |  |  |  |  |  |
|  |  |  |  |  |  |  |  |  |
|  |  |  |  |  |  |  |  |  |
|  |  |  |  |  |  |  |  |  |

| DATE | DISTANCE | TIME | PACE | HR | REST HR | RUN TYPE | SHOES | NOTES |
|------|----------|------|------|-----|---------|----------|-------|-------|

# RUNNING / JOGGING LOG

YEAR __________  MONTH __________

| DATE | DISTANCE | TIME | PACE | HR | REST HR | RUN TYPE | SHOES | NOTES |
|------|----------|------|------|-----|---------|----------|-------|-------|
|      |          |      |      |     |         |          |       |       |
|      |          |      |      |     |         |          |       |       |
|      |          |      |      |     |         |          |       |       |
|      |          |      |      |     |         |          |       |       |

| DATE | DISTANCE | TIME | PACE | HR | REST HR | RUN TYPE | SHOES | NOTES |
|------|----------|------|------|-----|---------|----------|-------|-------|
|      |          |      |      |     |         |          |       |       |

# RUNNING / JOGGING LOG

YEAR            MONTH

| DATE | DISTANCE | TIME | PACE | HR | REST HR | RUN TYPE | SHOES | NOTES |
|------|----------|------|------|----|---------|----------|-------|-------|
|      |          |      |      |    |         |          |       |       |

| DATE | DISTANCE | TIME | PACE | HR | REST HR | RUN TYPE | SHOES | NOTES |
|------|----------|------|------|----|---------|----------|-------|-------|
|      |          |      |      |    |         |          |       |       |

www.ingramcontent.com/pod-product-compliance
Lightning Source LLC
Chambersburg PA
CBHW070742250726
48662CB00004B/1617